RENAL DIET MEAL PLAN COOKBOOK

Delicious and Nutritious Recipes for Kidney Health

Dr Lily Morgan

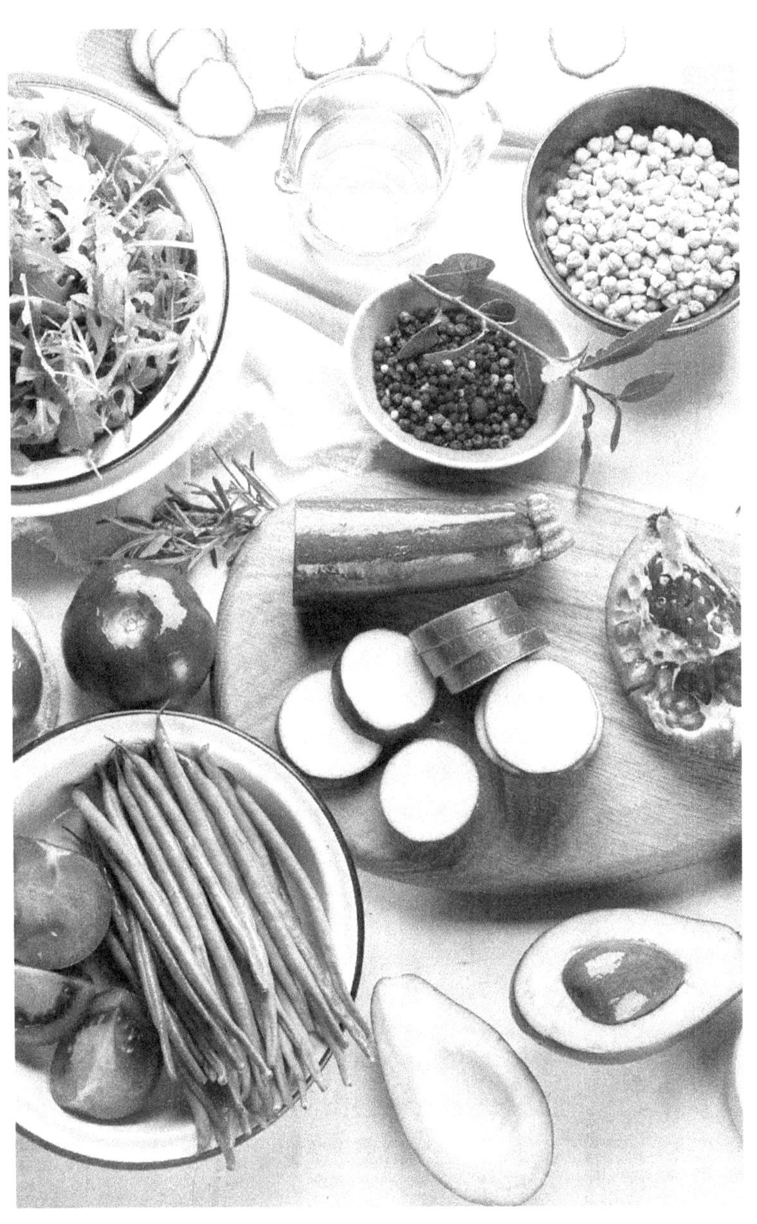

TABLE OF CONTENTS

Chapter 6: Desserts 81

INTRODUCTION

In the realm of nutrition and health, the renal diet stands as a specialized dietary approach with a profound impact on kidney health. It's not just a set of guidelines but a tailored way of eating designed to support and protect the intricate function of our kidneys.

The renal diet, primarily recommended for individuals with kidney conditions, places a strong emphasis on controlling the intake of certain nutrients, notably sodium, potassium, and phosphorus. By doing so, it aims to alleviate the burden on the kidneys and maintain a healthy balance of these elements in the body.

One of the key aspects of understanding the renal diet is recognizing that it's not a one-size-fits-all approach. It's tailored to an individual's specific needs, taking into account their kidney function, stage of kidney disease, and other health factors. This personalized approach makes it highly effective in managing kidney-related issues.

Now, let's delve into the benefits of adopting a renal-friendly diet. First and foremost, it plays a pivotal role in slowing down the progression of kidney disease. By meticulously controlling nutrient intake, it helps reduce the strain on the kidneys and potentially delay the need for dialysis or transplantation.

Moreover, a renal-friendly diet can aid in managing common complications of kidney disease, such as high blood pressure and fluid retention. By regulating sodium and fluid intake, it contributes to maintaining healthy blood pressure levels and preventing edema.

Another notable benefit is the preservation of bone health. Kidney disease often disrupts the balance of calcium and phosphorus in the body, potentially leading to bone issues. A renal diet, with its controlled phosphorus intake, helps safeguard bone health.

Lastly, the renal diet can enhance overall well-being by providing necessary nutrients while minimizing harm to the kidneys. It supports individuals in maintaining a fulfilling and nutritious diet even in the face of kidney-related challenges.

In summary, understanding the renal diet and embracing its principles can have a transformative impact on kidney health. This personalized dietary approach is not merely a set of restrictions but a path to maintaining kidney function, managing complications, and promoting well-being for those navigating the complexities of kidney disease.

Chapter 1: 30-Day Meal Plan

Week 1:

Day 1:

- Breakfast: Cinnamon Oatmeal Porridge
- Lunch: Quinoa and Chickpea Salad
- Dinner: Baked Cod with Lemon and Herbs
- Snacks: Guacamole with Veggie Sticks
- Dessert: Baked Apple with Cinnamon

Day 2:

- Breakfast: Veggie and Cheese Omelette
- Lunch: Turkey and Avocado Wrap
- Dinner: Stuffed Bell Peppers
- Snacks: Hummus and Pita Chips
- Dessert: Berry Sorbet

Day 3:

- Breakfast: Berry Breakfast Parfait
- Lunch: Caprese Salad with Balsamic Glaze
- Dinner: Teriyaki Tofu and Broccoli

- Snacks: Cottage Cheese with Pineapple
- Dessert: Chocolate Avocado Mousse

Day 4:

- Breakfast: Apple Cinnamon Quinoa Bowl
- Lunch: Lentil Soup
- Dinner: Beef and Vegetable Stir-Fry
- Snacks: Roasted Red Pepper Dip
- Dessert: Rice Pudding with Raisins

Day 5:

- Breakfast: Breakfast Smoothie
- Lunch: Chicken and Vegetable Stir-Fry
- Dinner: Mediterranean Baked Chicken
- Snacks: Fruit Salad
- Dessert: Peach and Almond Crumble

Day 6:

- Breakfast: Spinach and Mushroom Frittata
- Lunch: Tuna Salad with Greek Yogurt
- Dinner: Spaghetti Squash with Pesto
- Snacks: Greek Salad Skewers

- Dessert: Chia Seed Pudding

Day 7:

- Breakfast: Avocado Toast with Poached Egg
- Lunch: Spinach and Strawberry Salad
- Dinner: Grilled Salmon with Dill Sauce
- Snacks: Cucumber Slices with Tzatziki
- Dessert: Frozen Yogurt with Berries

Week 2:

Day 8:

- Breakfast: Creamy Rice Pudding
- Lunch: Black Bean and Corn Salad
- Dinner: Vegetarian Chili
- Snacks: Mixed Nuts
- Dessert: Watermelon and Mint Salad

Day 9:

- Breakfast: Sweet Potato Pancakes
- Lunch: Ratatouille
- Dinner: Lemon Garlic Shrimp Scampi
- Snacks: Deviled Eggs

- Dessert: Banana Ice Cream

Day 10:

- Breakfast: Greek Yogurt with Honey and Nuts
- Lunch: White Bean and Kale Soup
- Dinner: BBQ Pulled Chicken
- Snacks: Spinach and Artichoke Dip
- Dessert: Pistachio Biscotti

Day 11:

- Breakfast: Blueberry Buckwheat Pancakes
- Lunch: Grilled Chicken Caesar Salad
- Dinner: Spinach and Feta Stuffed Chicken Breast
- Snacks: Rice Cakes with Almond Butter
- Dessert: Mixed Berry Parfait

Day 12:

- Breakfast: Scrambled Eggs with Spinach
- Lunch: Minestrone Soup
- Dinner: Veggie Stir-Fried Rice
- Snacks: Caprese Skewers
- Dessert: Oatmeal Cookies

Day 13:

- Breakfast: Breakfast Burrito
- Lunch: Egg Salad
- Dinner: Baked Eggplant Parmesan
- Snacks: Salsa and Baked Tortilla Chips
- Dessert: Carrot Cake Bites

Day 14:

- Breakfast: Whole Grain Waffles
- Lunch: Mediterranean Couscous Salad
- Dinner: Pork Tenderloin with Apple Compote
- Snacks: Popcorn with Herbs
- Dessert: Pineapple Upside-Down Cake

Week 3:

Day 15:

- Breakfast: Almond Butter Toast
- Lunch: Salmon and Asparagus
- Dinner: Vegetarian Lasagna
- Snacks: Stuffed Mushrooms
- Dessert: Pumpkin Pie

Day 16:

- Breakfast: Muesli with Fresh Fruit
- Lunch: Mexican Bean Burrito Bowl
- Dinner: Lemon Butter Tilapia
- Snacks: Fruit Smoothie
- Dessert: Angel Food Cake with Berries

Day 17:

- Breakfast: Tofu Scramble
- Lunch: Broccoli and Cheddar Soup
- Dinner: Ratatouille Stuffed Zucchini
- Snacks: Sweet Potato Fries
- Dessert: Caramelized Bananas

Day 18:

- Breakfast: Banana Walnut Muffins
- Lunch: Shrimp and Quinoa Salad
- Dinner: Beef and Vegetable Kebabs
- Snacks: Baked Mozzarella Sticks
- Dessert: Chocolate-Dipped Strawberries

Day 19:

- Breakfast: Cinnamon Oatmeal Porridge
- Lunch: Quinoa and Chickpea Salad
- Dinner: Baked Cod with Lemon and Herbs
- Snacks: Guacamole with Veggie Sticks
- Dessert: Baked Apple with Cinnamon

Day 20:

- Breakfast: Veggie and Cheese Omelette
- Lunch: Turkey and Avocado Wrap
- Dinner: Stuffed Bell Peppers
- Snacks: Hummus and Pita Chips
- Dessert: Berry Sorbet

Day 21:

- Breakfast: Berry Breakfast Parfait
- Lunch: Caprese Salad with Balsamic Glaze
- Dinner: Teriyaki Tofu and Broccoli
- Snacks: Cottage Cheese with Pineapple
- Dessert: Chocolate Avocado Mousse

Day 22:

- Breakfast: Apple Cinnamon Quinoa Bowl
- Lunch: Lentil Soup
- Dinner: Beef and Vegetable Stir-Fry
- Snacks: Roasted Red Pepper Dip
- Dessert: Rice Pudding with Raisins

Day 23:

- Breakfast: Breakfast Smoothie
- Lunch: Chicken and Vegetable Stir-Fry
- Dinner: Mediterranean Baked Chicken
- Snacks: Fruit Salad
- Dessert: Peach and Almond Crumble

Day 24:

- Breakfast: Spinach and Mushroom Frittata
- Lunch: Tuna Salad with Greek Yogurt
- Dinner: Spaghetti Squash with Pesto
- Snacks: Greek Salad Skewers
- Dessert: Chia Seed Pudding

Day 25:

- Breakfast: Avocado Toast with Poached Egg
- Lunch: Spinach and Strawberry Salad
- Dinner: Grilled Salmon with Dill Sauce
- Snacks: Cucumber Slices with Tzatziki
- Dessert: Frozen Yogurt with Berries

Day 26:

- Breakfast: Creamy Rice Pudding
- Lunch: Black Bean and Corn Salad
- Dinner: Vegetarian Chili
- Snacks: Mixed Nuts
- Dessert: Watermelon and Mint Salad

Day 27:

- Breakfast: Sweet Potato Pancakes
- Lunch: Ratatouille
- Dinner: Lemon Garlic Shrimp Scampi
- Snacks: Deviled Eggs
- Dessert: Banana Ice Cream

Day 28:

- Breakfast: Greek Yogurt with Honey and Nuts
- Lunch: White Bean and Kale Soup
- Dinner: BBQ Pulled Chicken
- Snacks: Spinach and Artichoke Dip
- Dessert: Pistachio Biscotti

Day 29:

- Breakfast: Blueberry Buckwheat Pancakes
- Lunch: Grilled Chicken Caesar Salad
- Dinner: Spinach and Feta Stuffed Chicken Breast
- Snacks: Rice Cakes with Almond Butter
- Dessert: Mixed Berry Parfait

Day 30:

- Breakfast: Scrambled Eggs with Spinach
- Lunch: Minestrone Soup
- Dinner: Veggie Stir-Fried Rice
- Snacks: Caprese Skewers
- Dessert: Oatmeal Cookies

This completes your 30-day meal plan using the provided recipes. Enjoy a diverse range of delicious meals for breakfast, lunch, dinner, snacks, and dessert over the course of a month.

In this chapter, we've curated a delightful collection of kidney-friendly breakfast recipes. These dishes are not only delicious but also designed to support your renal health. You'll find a wide range of flavors and textures, ensuring that your mornings are filled with satisfaction and nourishment.

Cinnamon Oatmeal Porridge

Ingredients:

- 1/2 cup of rolled oats
- 1 cup of almond milk
- 1/2 teaspoon of cinnamon
- 1 tablespoon of honey
- Sliced banana (optional)

Instructions:

1. In a saucepan, combine oats and almond milk.
2. Add cinnamon and heat on medium, stirring occasionally until it thickens.

3. Drizzle with honey and top with sliced banana if desired.

Veggie and Cheese Omelette

Ingredients:

- 2 eggs
- 2 tablespoons of diced bell peppers
- 2 tablespoons of diced tomatoes
- 2 tablespoons of shredded low-sodium cheese
- Salt and pepper to taste

Instructions:

1. Whisk the eggs in a bowl and season with salt and pepper.
2. Heat a non-stick pan, add the vegetables, and pour the whisked eggs over them.
3. Cook until the edges set, then sprinkle cheese over one half and fold the omelette in half.
4. Cook until the cheese melts and serve.

Berry Breakfast Parfait

Ingredients:

- 1/2 cup of Greek yogurt
- 1/4 cup of mixed berries (strawberries, blueberries, raspberries)
- 2 tablespoons of granola

Instructions:

1. In a glass or bowl, layer Greek yogurt, mixed berries, and granola.
2. Repeat the layers as desired.
3. Enjoy this delightful parfait that's rich in antioxidants and protein.

Apple Cinnamon Quinoa Bowl

Ingredients:

- 1/2 cup of cooked quinoa
- 1/2 apple, chopped
- 1/4 teaspoon of cinnamon
- 1 tablespoon of chopped nuts (e.g., almonds or walnuts)

Instructions:

1. In a bowl, combine cooked quinoa and chopped apple.
2. Sprinkle with cinnamon and top with chopped nuts.
3. Mix well and savor the delightful blend of flavors.

Breakfast Smoothie

Ingredients:

- 1/2 cup of frozen mixed berries
- 1/2 banana
- 1/2 cup of spinach
- 1/2 cup of unsweetened almond milk
- 1 tablespoon of chia seeds

Instructions:

1. Blend all the ingredients until smooth.
2. Pour into a glass and enjoy a refreshing and nutritious breakfast smoothie.

Spinach and Mushroom Frittata

Ingredients:

- 2 eggs
- 1/4 cup of chopped spinach
- 1/4 cup of sliced mushrooms
- 1 tablespoon of grated Parmesan cheese
- Salt and pepper to taste

Instructions:

1. Whisk the eggs in a bowl and season with salt and pepper.
2. Heat a non-stick pan, add spinach and mushrooms, then pour the whisked eggs over them.
3. Sprinkle with Parmesan cheese.
4. Cook until the edges set, then place under the broiler until the top is golden.
5. Slice and serve this flavorful frittata.

Avocado Toast with Poached Egg

Ingredients:

- 1 slice of whole-grain bread

- 1/2 ripe avocado

- 1 poached egg

- Salt and pepper to taste

Instructions:

1. Toast the whole-grain bread.

2. Mash the ripe avocado and spread it on the toast.

3. Top with a poached egg, and season with salt and pepper.

4. A perfect combination of creamy and savory flavors.

Creamy Rice Pudding

Ingredients:

- 1/2 cup of cooked white rice

- 1/2 cup of low-fat milk

- 1/2 teaspoon of vanilla extract

- 1 tablespoon of honey

- A pinch of ground cinnamon

Instructions:

1. In a saucepan, combine cooked rice and milk.

2. Heat on low, stirring until it thickens.

3. Stir in vanilla extract and honey.

4. Sprinkle with ground cinnamon for added flavor.

Sweet Potato Pancakes

Ingredients:

- 1/2 cup of grated sweet potato

- 1 egg

- 2 tablespoons of whole-wheat flour

- 1/4 teaspoon of cinnamon

- 1/4 teaspoon of nutmeg

Instructions:

1. In a bowl, combine grated sweet potato, egg, flour, cinnamon, and nutmeg.

2. Heat a non-stick pan and drop spoonfuls of the mixture to make pancakes.

3. Cook until golden brown on each side.

4. Serve these nutritious and tasty pancakes.

Greek Yogurt with Honey and Nuts

Ingredients:

- 1/2 cup of Greek yogurt

- 1 tablespoon of honey

- 1 tablespoon of chopped nuts (e.g., almonds or walnuts)

Instructions:

1. In a bowl, scoop Greek yogurt.
2. Drizzle with honey and sprinkle chopped nuts on top.
3. A simple yet delightful breakfast option.

Blueberry Buckwheat Pancakes

Ingredients:

- 1/2 cup of buckwheat flour

- 1/4 cup of fresh blueberries

- 1 egg

- 1/2 cup of almond milk

- 1/4 teaspoon of vanilla extract

Instructions:

1. In a bowl, combine buckwheat flour, blueberries, egg, almond milk, and vanilla extract.
2. Heat a non-stick pan and make pancakes from the mixture.
3. Cook until they're golden and blueberries burst.

Scrambled Eggs with Spinach

Ingredients:

- 2 eggs
- 1/2 cup of chopped spinach
- 1/4 cup of diced tomatoes
- Salt and pepper to taste

Instructions:

1. Whisk the eggs in a bowl and season with salt and pepper.
2. Heat a pan, add spinach and tomatoes, and pour in the eggs.
3. Scramble until cooked to your liking.
4. A nutritious and flavorful breakfast.

Breakfast Burrito

Ingredients:

- 1 whole-wheat tortilla
- 1 scrambled egg
- 1/4 cup of black beans
- Salsa for topping

Instructions:

1. Place scrambled egg and black beans on the tortilla.
2. Roll it up and top with salsa.
3. A savory breakfast on the go.

Whole Grain Waffles

Ingredients:

- 1 whole-grain waffle
- 1/4 cup of low-sugar fruit compote (e.g., apple or berry)
- Greek yogurt for topping

Instructions:

1. Toast the whole-grain waffle.

2. Top with fruit compote and a dollop of Greek yogurt.

3. A delightful waffle with a fruity twist.

Almond Butter Toast

Ingredients:

- 1 slice of whole-grain bread

- 1 tablespoon of almond butter

- Sliced bananas for topping

Instructions:

1. Toast the whole-grain bread.

2. Spread almond butter and top with sliced bananas.

3. A quick and wholesome option.

Muesli with Fresh Fruit

Ingredients:

- 1/2 cup of muesli

- Sliced fresh fruit (e.g., strawberries, kiwi, or melon)

- Low-fat milk or yogurt for serving

Instructions:

1. In a bowl, combine muesli and fresh fruit.

2. Add low-fat milk or yogurt for a nutritious bowl.

Tofu Scramble

Ingredients:

- 1/2 cup of crumbled tofu

- 1/4 cup of diced bell peppers

- 1/4 cup of spinach

- Turmeric for color and flavor

- Salt and pepper to taste

Instructions:

1. In a pan, sauté bell peppers and spinach.

2. Add crumbled tofu and season with turmeric, salt, and pepper.

3. Cook until heated through, and serve this protein-packed scramble.

Banana Walnut Muffins

Ingredients:

- 1 ripe banana, mashed
- 1/4 cup of chopped walnuts
- 1/4 cup of whole-wheat flour
- 1 egg
- 1/4 cup of Greek yogurt

Instructions:

1. In a bowl, combine mashed banana, chopped walnuts, whole-wheat flour, egg, and Greek yogurt.
2. Mix until smooth and pour into muffin cups.
3. Bake until golden and enjoy these delectable muffins.

Chapter 3: Lunch Recipes

In Chapter 3, we're diving into a delightful array of lunch recipes that are not only kidney-friendly but also packed with flavor and nutrition. These dishes provide a perfect midday boost to keep you energized and satisfied. Below, you'll find a selection of these recipes, each thoughtfully crafted to fit your renal diet needs.

Quinoa and Chickpea Salad

Ingredients:

- 1 cup cooked quinoa
- 1 can chickpeas, drained and rinsed
- 1 cup diced cucumber
- 1 cup diced red bell pepper
- 1/2 cup chopped fresh parsley
- 1/4 cup olive oil
- 2 tablespoons lemon juice
- Salt and pepper to taste

Instructions:

1. In a large bowl, combine quinoa, chickpeas, cucumber, red bell pepper, and fresh parsley.
2. In a separate small bowl, whisk together olive oil and lemon juice.
3. Drizzle the dressing over the salad and toss to combine.
4. Season with salt and pepper to taste.
5. Chill in the refrigerator for at least 30 minutes before serving.

Turkey and Avocado Wrap

Ingredients:

- 4 whole-grain tortillas
- 2 cups cooked turkey breast, thinly sliced
- 2 ripe avocados, sliced
- 1 cup fresh spinach leaves
- 1/4 cup low-fat mayonnaise
- 2 tablespoons Dijon mustard

Instructions:

1. Lay out the tortillas and spread a thin layer of mayonnaise and Dijon mustard on each.
2. Place turkey slices, avocado, and spinach in the center of each tortilla.
3. Roll the tortillas tightly, folding in the sides as you go.
4. Slice in half and serve.

Caprese Salad with Balsamic Glaze

Ingredients:

- 4 ripe tomatoes, sliced
- 1 cup fresh mozzarella cheese, sliced
- 1/2 cup fresh basil leaves
- 3 tablespoons balsamic glaze
- Salt and black pepper to taste

Instructions:

1. Arrange tomato, mozzarella, and basil slices on a platter.
2. Drizzle balsamic glaze over the top.
3. Season with salt and black pepper.

4. Serve immediately as a refreshing salad.

Lentil Soup

Ingredients:

- 1 cup dried green lentils
- 6 cups low-sodium vegetable broth
- 1 onion, diced
- 2 carrots, diced
- 2 celery stalks, diced
- 2 cloves garlic, minced
- 1 teaspoon cumin
- 1/2 teaspoon smoked paprika
- Salt and pepper to taste

Instructions:

1. Rinse the lentils under cold water and drain.
2. In a large pot, sauté the onion, carrots, celery, and garlic until softened.
3. Add lentils, vegetable broth, cumin, and smoked paprika.
4. Simmer for about 30-40 minutes until lentils are tender.

5. Season with salt and pepper and serve hot.

Chicken and Vegetable Stir-Fry

Ingredients:

- 2 boneless, skinless chicken breasts, sliced
- 2 cups broccoli florets
- 1 red bell pepper, sliced
- 1 cup snow peas
- 1/4 cup low-sodium stir-fry sauce
- 2 tablespoons vegetable oil
- 2 cups cooked brown rice

Instructions:

1. Heat vegetable oil in a large skillet over medium-high heat.
2. Add chicken slices and stir-fry until cooked through.
3. Add broccoli, bell pepper, and snow peas; stir-fry for a few minutes.
4. Pour in the stir-fry sauce and continue cooking until the vegetables are tender.
5. Serve over cooked brown rice.

Tuna Salad with Greek Yogurt

Ingredients:

- 2 cans of low-sodium tuna, drained
- 1/2 cup Greek yogurt
- 1/4 cup diced red onion
- 1/4 cup diced celery
- 1 tablespoon Dijon mustard
- Salt and pepper to taste

Instructions:

1. In a bowl, combine drained tuna, Greek yogurt, red onion, celery, and Dijon mustard.
2. Mix until well combined.
3. Season with salt and pepper.
4. Serve as a salad or in a sandwich.

Spinach and Strawberry Salad

Ingredients:

- 4 cups fresh spinach leaves
- 1 cup sliced strawberries
- 1/4 cup crumbled feta cheese

- 1/4 cup chopped walnuts
- Balsamic vinaigrette dressing

Instructions:

1. In a salad bowl, combine fresh spinach, sliced strawberries, feta cheese, and walnuts.
2. Drizzle with balsamic vinaigrette dressing to taste.
3. Toss gently and serve as a refreshing salad.

Black Bean and Corn Salad

Ingredients:

- 1 can black beans, drained and rinsed
- 1 cup frozen corn, thawed
- 1 red bell pepper, diced
- 1/4 cup chopped cilantro
- 2 tablespoons lime juice
- 1 tablespoon olive oil
- Salt and black pepper to taste

Instructions:

1. In a bowl, combine black beans, corn, red bell pepper, and cilantro.

2. In a separate small bowl, whisk together lime juice and olive oil.

3. Drizzle the dressing over the salad and toss.

4. Season with salt and black pepper.

5. Serve as a zesty and protein-rich salad.

Ratatouille

Ingredients:

- 1 eggplant, diced
- 1 zucchini, diced
- 1 yellow squash, diced
- 1 red bell pepper, diced
- 1 onion, diced
- 2 cloves garlic, minced
- 1 can diced tomatoes
- 2 tablespoons olive oil
- 1 teaspoon dried basil
- Salt and black pepper to taste

Instructions:

1. In a large pot, heat olive oil and sauté the onion and garlic.

2. Add eggplant, zucchini, yellow squash, and red bell pepper.

3. Stir in diced tomatoes and dried basil.

4. Simmer until the vegetables are tender.

5. Season with salt and black pepper and serve.

White Bean and Kale Soup

Ingredients:

- 2 cups cooked white beans
- 4 cups vegetable broth
- 2 cups chopped kale
- 1 onion, diced
- 2 cloves garlic, minced
- 1 teaspoon dried thyme
- Salt and black pepper to taste

Instructions:

1. In a large pot, sauté the onion and garlic until translucent.

2. Add cooked white beans, vegetable broth, and dried thyme.

3. Simmer for about 15 minutes.

4. Stir in the chopped kale and cook until wilted.

5. Season with salt and black pepper and serve hot.

Grilled Chicken Caesar Salad

Ingredients:

- 2 boneless, skinless chicken breasts
- 4 cups chopped romaine lettuce
- 1/4 cup grated Parmesan cheese
- Whole-grain croutons
- Low-sodium Caesar dressing

Instructions:

1. Grill the chicken breasts until cooked through.

2. Slice the grilled chicken.

3. In a bowl, combine romaine lettuce, grated Parmesan, and whole-grain croutons.

4. Add the sliced chicken.

5. Drizzle with low-sodium Caesar dressing and toss to coat.

Minestrone Soup

Ingredients:

- 6 cups low-sodium vegetable broth
- 1 cup chopped carrots
- 1 cup diced celery
- 1 onion, diced
- 2 cloves garlic, minced
- 1 cup small pasta
- 1 can kidney beans, drained and rinsed
- 1 can diced tomatoes
- 1 teaspoon Italian seasoning
- Salt and black pepper to taste

Instructions:

1. In a large pot, sauté the onion and garlic until softened.
2. Add vegetable broth, carrots, celery, small pasta, kidney beans, diced tomatoes, and Italian seasoning.
3. Simmer for about 20 minutes or until the vegetables are tender.
4. Season with salt and black pepper and serve hot.

Egg Salad

Ingredients:

- 6 hard-boiled eggs, chopped
- 1/4 cup low-fat mayonnaise
- 1 teaspoon Dijon mustard
- 1/4 cup chopped celery
- 1/4 cup chopped red onion
- Salt and black pepper to taste

Instructions:

1. In a bowl, combine chopped hard-boiled eggs, low-fat mayonnaise, and Dijon mustard.
2. Stir in chopped celery and red onion.
3. Season with salt and black pepper.
4. Serve as a delicious sandwich or salad.

Mediterranean Couscous Salad

Ingredients:

- 1 cup cooked couscous
- 1 cucumber, diced
- 1 cup cherry tomatoes, halved

- 1/4 cup chopped fresh parsley
- 1/4 cup feta cheese
- 2 tablespoons olive oil
- 1 tablespoon lemon juice
- Salt and black pepper to taste

Instructions:

1. In a large bowl, combine cooked couscous, diced cucumber, cherry tomatoes, fresh parsley, and feta cheese.
2. In a separate small bowl, whisk together olive oil and lemon juice.
3. Drizzle the dressing over the salad and toss.
4. Season with salt and black pepper.
5. Serve as a light and refreshing salad.

Salmon and Asparagus

Ingredients:

- 4 salmon fillets
- 1 bunch asparagus, trimmed
- 2 tablespoons olive oil
- 1 lemon, sliced

- 1 teaspoon dried dill

- Salt and black pepper to taste

Instructions:

1. Preheat your oven to 375°F (190°C).

2. Place salmon fillets and asparagus on a baking sheet.

3. Drizzle with olive oil and sprinkle with dried dill.

4. Season with salt and black pepper.

5. Top with lemon slices.

6. Bake for about 15-20 minutes or until salmon flakes easily.

Mexican Bean Burrito Bowl

Ingredients:

- 1 cup cooked brown rice

- 1 can black beans, drained and rinsed

- 1 cup corn kernels

- 1 cup diced tomatoes

- 1/4 cup chopped cilantro

- 1 teaspoon cumin

- 1/2 teaspoon chili powder

- Salt and black pepper to taste

Instructions:

1. In a bowl, combine cooked brown rice, black beans, corn kernels, diced tomatoes, and chopped cilantro.
2. Season with cumin, chili powder, salt, and black pepper.
3. Toss to mix.
4. Serve as a tasty burrito bowl.

Broccoli and Cheddar Soup

Ingredients:

- 4 cups low-sodium vegetable broth
- 4 cups chopped broccoli florets
- 1 onion, diced
- 2 cloves garlic, minced
- 1 cup grated low-fat cheddar cheese
- Salt and black pepper to taste

Instructions:

1. In a large pot, sauté the onion and garlic until softened.
2. Add vegetable broth and broccoli florets.

3. Simmer for about 20 minutes or until the broccoli is tender.

4. Use an immersion blender to puree the soup.

5. Stir in grated low-fat cheddar cheese.

6. Season with salt and black pepper and serve hot.

Shrimp and Quinoa Salad

Ingredients:

- 1 cup cooked quinoa
- 1 lb cooked and peeled shrimp
- 1 cup cherry tomatoes, halved
- 1/4 cup chopped fresh cilantro
- 2 tablespoons olive oil
- 2 tablespoons lime juice
- Salt and black pepper to taste

Instructions:

1. In a bowl, combine cooked quinoa, cooked shrimp, cherry tomatoes, and fresh cilantro.

2. In a separate small bowl, whisk together olive oil and lime juice.

3. Drizzle the dressing over the salad and toss.

4. Season with salt and black pepper.

5. Serve as a light and protein-packed salad.

In this chapter, we've curated a delightful selection of dinner recipes designed to be both kidney-friendly and delicious. From succulent meats to satisfying vegetarian options, you're sure to find a dinner that suits your taste and dietary requirements.

Baked Cod with Lemon and Herbs

Ingredients:

- 4 cod fillets
- 2 lemons
- Fresh herbs (e.g., rosemary, thyme)
- Olive oil
- Salt and pepper to taste

Instructions:

1. Preheat the oven to 375°F (190°C).
2. Place cod fillets on a baking sheet.
3. Drizzle with olive oil, then season with salt, pepper, and freshly squeezed lemon juice.

4. Sprinkle fresh herbs on top.

5. Bake for 15-20 minutes or until the cod is flaky and cooked through.

Stuffed Bell Peppers

Ingredients:

- 4 bell peppers
- 1 cup cooked rice
- 1 lb lean ground beef or turkey
- 1 can diced tomatoes
- 1 onion, chopped
- 1 cup shredded low-fat cheese
- Spices (e.g., oregano, basil)

Instructions:

1. Cut the tops off the bell peppers and remove seeds.

2. In a skillet, brown the ground meat with onions.

3. Add diced tomatoes and spices. Mix with cooked rice.

4. Stuff the bell peppers with the mixture.

5. Top with shredded cheese and bake at 350°F (175°C) for 25-30 minutes.

Teriyaki Tofu and Broccoli

Ingredients:

- 1 block of firm tofu, cubed
- 2 cups broccoli florets
- 1/2 cup low-sodium teriyaki sauce
- 2 cloves garlic, minced
- 1 tablespoon sesame oil
- Cooked brown rice

Instructions:

1. In a pan, sauté tofu in sesame oil until lightly browned.
2. Add minced garlic and broccoli. Stir-fry until tender.
3. Pour teriyaki sauce over tofu and broccoli. Cook until heated through.
4. Serve over cooked brown rice.

Beef and Vegetable Stir-Fry

Ingredients:

- 1 lb lean beef, thinly sliced

- Mixed vegetables (e.g., bell peppers, broccoli, carrots)
- 1/4 cup low-sodium soy sauce
- 2 cloves garlic, minced
- 1 tablespoon vegetable oil
- Cooked brown rice

Instructions:

1. In a wok or large skillet, heat oil and sauté garlic.
2. Add beef and stir-fry until browned. Remove from pan.
3. Stir-fry mixed vegetables until crisp-tender.
4. Return beef to the pan, add soy sauce, and cook briefly.
5. Serve over cooked brown rice.

Mediterranean Baked Chicken

Ingredients:

- 4 boneless, skinless chicken breasts
- 1 lemon
- 2 cloves garlic, minced
- 1 teaspoon dried oregano

- 1/4 cup olive oil

- Salt and pepper to taste

Instructions:

1. Preheat the oven to 375°F (190°C).

2. Place chicken breasts in a baking dish.

3. Squeeze lemon juice over chicken, then drizzle with olive oil.

4. Sprinkle minced garlic, dried oregano, salt, and pepper.

5. Bake for 25-30 minutes or until chicken is cooked through.

Spaghetti Squash with Pesto

Ingredients:

- 1 spaghetti squash

- 1/2 cup basil pesto

- Cherry tomatoes, halved

- Grated Parmesan cheese

Instructions:

1. Preheat the oven to 375°F (190°C).

2. Cut spaghetti squash in half and remove seeds.

3. Place squash halves cut side down on a baking sheet and bake for 40 minutes.

4. Scrape out the "spaghetti" with a fork.

5. Toss with pesto, cherry tomatoes, and top with Parmesan.

Grilled Salmon with Dill Sauce

Ingredients:

- 4 salmon fillets
- 1/4 cup plain Greek yogurt
- Fresh dill, chopped
- Lemon juice
- Salt and pepper to taste

Instructions:

1. Preheat the grill to medium-high heat.

2. Season salmon with salt, pepper, and lemon juice.

3. Grill salmon for 4-5 minutes per side.

4. Mix Greek yogurt, chopped dill, and a squeeze of lemon for the sauce.

5. Serve salmon with dill sauce.

Vegetarian Chili

Ingredients:

- 1 can kidney beans
- 1 can black beans
- 1 can diced tomatoes
- 1 onion, chopped
- 1 bell pepper, chopped
- Chili powder and cumin to taste

Instructions:

1. In a large pot, sauté onion and bell pepper until tender.
2. Add kidney beans, black beans, and diced tomatoes.
3. Season with chili powder and cumin.
4. Simmer for 20-30 minutes, stirring occasionally.

Lemon Garlic Shrimp Scampi

Ingredients:

- 1 lb large shrimp, peeled and deveined
- 3 cloves garlic, minced
- 2 tablespoons lemon juice

- 2 tablespoons unsalted butter

- Fresh parsley, chopped

- Cooked whole wheat pasta

Instructions:

1. In a pan, melt butter and add minced garlic. Sauté for a minute.

2. Add shrimp and cook until pink, about 2-3 minutes per side.

3. Stir in lemon juice and chopped parsley.

4. Serve over cooked whole wheat pasta.

BBQ Pulled Chicken

Ingredients:

- 1 lb boneless, skinless chicken breasts

- 1 cup low-sodium barbecue sauce

- 1/2 cup low-sodium chicken broth

- 1 onion, chopped

- Whole wheat buns

Instructions:

1. Place chicken breasts in a slow cooker.

2. Mix barbecue sauce, chicken broth, and chopped onion.

3. Pour the mixture over the chicken and cook on low for 6-8 hours.

4. Shred the chicken and serve on whole wheat buns.

Spinach and Feta Stuffed Chicken Breast

Ingredients:

- 4 boneless, skinless chicken breasts
- 1 cup frozen chopped spinach, thawed and drained
- 1/2 cup crumbled feta cheese
- 1 teaspoon garlic powder
- Salt and pepper to taste

Instructions:

1. Preheat the oven to 375°F (190°C).

2. Slice a pocket into each chicken breast.

3. Mix spinach, feta, garlic powder, salt, and pepper.

4. Stuff the chicken breasts with the mixture.

5. Bake for 25-30 minutes or until chicken is cooked through.

Veggie Stir-Fried Rice

Ingredients:

- 2 cups cooked brown rice
- Mixed vegetables (e.g., carrots, peas, bell peppers)
- 2 eggs, beaten
- Low-sodium soy sauce

Instructions:

1. In a pan, scramble the eggs and set aside.
2. Stir-fry mixed vegetables in the same pan.
3. Add cooked brown rice and eggs.
4. Drizzle with low-sodium soy sauce and toss until heated through.

Baked Eggplant Parmesan

Ingredients:

- 2 large eggplants
- 2 cups marinara sauce

- 1 cup shredded mozzarella cheese
- 1/2 cup grated Parmesan cheese
- Fresh basil leaves

Instructions:

1. Preheat the oven to 375°F (190°C).
2. Slice eggplants into rounds.
3. Layer eggplant slices, marinara sauce, and cheeses in a baking dish.
4. Repeat the layers and finish with cheese on top.
5. Bake for 25-30 minutes until cheese is bubbly and eggplant is tender.
6. Garnish with fresh basil leaves.

Pork Tenderloin with Apple Compote

Ingredients:

- 2 pork tenderloins
- 2 apples, peeled and chopped
- 1/4 cup apple juice
- 1/4 cup brown sugar

- Cinnamon and nutmeg to taste

Instructions:

1. Preheat the oven to 375°F (190°C).
2. Season pork tenderloins with cinnamon and nutmeg.
3. Place in a baking dish.
4. In a saucepan, cook apples, apple juice, and brown sugar until soft.
5. Spoon the compote over the pork and bake for 25-30 minutes.

Vegetarian Lasagna

Ingredients:

- Whole wheat lasagna noodles
- 1 cup part-skim ricotta cheese
- 2 cups chopped spinach
- 1 cup sliced mushrooms
- Low-sodium tomato sauce
- Part-skim mozzarella cheese

Instructions:

1. Cook lasagna noodles according to package instructions.
2. Layer noodles with ricotta cheese, spinach, mushrooms, and tomato sauce.
3. Repeat layers and top with mozzarella cheese.
4. Bake at 375°F (190°C) for 30-35 minutes.

Lemon Butter Tilapia

Ingredients:

- 4 tilapia fillets
- 1 lemon
- 2 tablespoons unsalted butter
- Fresh parsley, chopped
- Salt and pepper to taste

Instructions:

1. Preheat the oven to 375°F (190°C).
2. Place tilapia fillets in a baking dish.
3. Drizzle with melted butter and lemon juice.
4. Season with salt, pepper, and sprinkle with chopped parsley.

5. Bake for 15-20 minutes or until tilapia flakes easily.

Ratatouille Stuffed Zucchini

Ingredients:

- 4 large zucchinis
- 2 cups ratatouille (mixed vegetables and tomato sauce)
- 1/2 cup shredded low-fat cheese

Instructions:

1. Cut zucchinis in half lengthwise and scoop out the centers.
2. Fill each zucchini half with ratatouille.
3. Sprinkle with shredded cheese.
4. Bake at 375°F (190°C) for 20-25 minutes.

Beef and Vegetable Kebabs

Ingredients:

- Lean beef chunks
- Bell peppers, onions, and zucchini, cut into chunks
- Low-sodium marinade

- Wooden skewers (soaked in water)

Instructions:

1. Thread beef and vegetables onto skewers.

2. Marinate the kebabs in low-sodium sauce.

3. Grill until beef is cooked and vegetables are tender.

Chapter 5: Snacks and Appetizers

In Chapter 5, we dive into a world of delightful snacking and appetizers designed to tantalize your taste buds while keeping your renal diet on track. These savory, crunchy, and flavorful options are perfect for satisfying those in-between meal cravings. Get ready to explore a variety of delectable choices.

Guacamole with Veggie Sticks

Ingredients:

- 2 ripe avocados
- 1 small onion, finely chopped
- 1 clove garlic, minced
- 1 tomato, diced
- 1 lime, juiced
- Salt and pepper to taste
- Assorted veggie sticks (carrots, celery, bell peppers)

Instructions:

1. Cut the avocados in half, remove the pits, and scoop the flesh into a bowl.

2. Mash the avocado with a fork and combine it with chopped onion, garlic, and diced tomato.

3. Add lime juice, salt, and pepper, then mix well.

4. Serve with a platter of assorted veggie sticks for dipping.

Hummus and Pita Chips

Ingredients:

*   1 can of chickpeas, drained and rinsed
*   2 cloves garlic, minced
*   3 tablespoons tahini
*   2 tablespoons lemon juice
*   2 tablespoons olive oil
*   1/2 teaspoon cumin
*   Salt and paprika to taste
*   Whole-grain pita chips

Instructions:

1. In a food processor, blend chickpeas, garlic, tahini, lemon juice, olive oil, cumin, salt, and paprika until smooth.

2. Serve the hummus with whole-grain pita chips for dipping.

Cottage Cheese with Pineapple

Ingredients:

- Low-fat cottage cheese
- Fresh pineapple chunks

Instructions:

1. Simply spoon low-fat cottage cheese into a bowl.

2. Top with fresh pineapple chunks for a refreshing and creamy snack.

Roasted Red Pepper Dip

Ingredients:

- 2 red bell peppers
- 1/4 cup plain Greek yogurt

- 1 clove garlic, minced

- 1 tablespoon olive oil

- Salt and pepper to taste

- Whole-grain crackers or veggie sticks

Instructions:

1. Roast red bell peppers until the skin is charred. Peel, remove seeds, and chop.

2. In a blender, combine roasted red peppers, Greek yogurt, minced garlic, olive oil, salt, and pepper. Blend until smooth.

3. Serve with whole-grain crackers or veggie sticks.

Fruit Salad

Ingredients:

- A variety of fresh fruits (e.g., strawberries, blueberries, melon, grapes)

- A squeeze of fresh lime juice

Instructions:

1. Wash and cut fruits into bite-sized pieces.

2. Toss them together in a bowl and add a squeeze of fresh lime juice for a zesty twist.

Greek Salad Skewers

Ingredients:

- Cherry tomatoes
- Cucumber, cut into chunks
- Kalamata olives
- Feta cheese, cubed
- Fresh basil leaves
- Balsamic glaze

Instructions:

1. Thread cherry tomatoes, cucumber chunks, Kalamata olives, feta cheese, and fresh basil leaves onto skewers.
2. Drizzle with balsamic glaze for a burst of Mediterranean flavors.

Cucumber Slices with Tzatziki

Ingredients:

- Cucumber, thinly sliced
- Tzatziki sauce

Instructions:

1. Arrange thin cucumber slices on a plate.
2. Serve with tzatziki sauce for a cooling and refreshing snack.

Mixed Nuts

Ingredients:

- A variety of unsalted mixed nuts (e.g., almonds, walnuts, cashews)

Instructions:

1. Simply serve a handful of mixed nuts for a satisfying and nutritious snack.

Deviled Eggs

Ingredients:

- Hard-boiled eggs, halved

- Egg yolks

- Mayonnaise

- Dijon mustard

- Paprika

- Chopped chives

Instructions:

1. Remove egg yolks and mix them with mayonnaise, Dijon mustard, and a pinch of paprika.

2. Spoon the yolk mixture back into egg white halves and garnish with chopped chives.

Spinach and Artichoke Dip

Ingredients:

- 1 cup frozen spinach, thawed and drained

- 1 cup canned artichoke hearts, drained and chopped

- 1 cup Greek yogurt

- 1/4 cup grated Parmesan cheese

- 1/4 cup low-fat cream cheese

- 1 clove garlic, minced

- Salt and pepper to taste

- Whole-grain pita chips or veggie sticks

Instructions:

1. In a bowl, mix thawed spinach, chopped artichoke hearts, Greek yogurt, grated Parmesan cheese, low-fat cream cheese, minced garlic, salt, and pepper.

2. Serve with whole-grain pita chips or veggie sticks.

Rice Cakes with Almond Butter

Ingredients:

- Whole-grain rice cakes

- Almond butter

Instructions:

1. Spread a layer of almond butter on whole-grain rice cakes for a crunchy and nutty snack.

Caprese Skewers

Ingredients:

- Cherry tomatoes
- Fresh mozzarella balls
- Fresh basil leaves
- Balsamic glaze

Instructions:

1. Thread cherry tomatoes, fresh mozzarella balls, and fresh basil leaves onto skewers.
2. Drizzle with balsamic glaze for a taste of Italy.

Salsa and Baked Tortilla Chips

Ingredients:

- Low-sodium salsa
- Baked whole-grain tortilla chips

Instructions:

1. Serve low-sodium salsa with baked whole-grain tortilla chips for a zesty and guilt-free snack.

Popcorn with Herbs

Ingredients:

- Air-popped popcorn
- Olive oil
- Dried herbs (e.g., rosemary, thyme, oregano)
- Salt and pepper to taste

Instructions:

1. Drizzle air-popped popcorn with a bit of olive oil, dried herbs, salt, and pepper for a flavorful popcorn experience.

Stuffed Mushrooms

Ingredients:

- Fresh button mushrooms
- Cream cheese
- Garlic, minced
- Fresh parsley, chopped
- Grated Parmesan cheese

Instructions:

1. Remove stems from mushrooms and mix them with cream cheese, minced garlic, fresh parsley, and grated Parmesan cheese.

2. Stuff the mushroom caps with the mixture and bake until golden brown.

Fruit Smoothie

Ingredients:

- Your choice of fruits (e.g., bananas, berries, mango)
- Greek yogurt
- Ice
- Honey (optional)

Instructions:

1. Blend your favorite fruits with Greek yogurt, ice, and honey (if desired) for a refreshing and nutritious fruit smoothie.

Sweet Potato Fries

Ingredients:

- Sweet potatoes, cut into fries
- Olive oil
- Seasonings (e.g., paprika, garlic powder, salt)

Instructions:

1. Toss sweet potato fries with olive oil and your choice of seasonings.
2. Bake until crispy and serve as a healthier alternative to traditional fries.

Baked Mozzarella Sticks

Ingredients:

- Part-skim mozzarella cheese sticks
- Whole-grain breadcrumbs
- Italian seasoning
- Marinara sauce for dipping

Instructions:

1. Coat mozzarella sticks with whole-grain breadcrumbs mixed with Italian seasoning.
2. Bake until golden and serve with marinara sauce for a cheesy and satisfying snack.

These desserts are not only delicious but also tailored to support your kidney health. From the simplicity of a Baked Apple with Cinnamon to the richness of Chocolate Avocado Mousse, you'll find a treat for every occasion and craving. Let's dive into these delectable creations.

Baked Apple with Cinnamon

Ingredients:

- 4 apples
- 1 tablespoon ground cinnamon
- 2 tablespoons brown sugar (or sugar substitute)

Instructions:

1. Preheat your oven to 375°F (190°C).
2. Core the apples, leaving the bottoms intact.
3. In a small bowl, combine the cinnamon and brown sugar.
4. Sprinkle the cinnamon-sugar mixture inside each apple.

5. Place the apples in a baking dish and bake for 25-30 minutes until tender.

6. Serve warm, and enjoy the comforting aroma of baked apples.

Berry Sorbet

Ingredients:

- 2 cups mixed berries (strawberries, blueberries, raspberries)
- 1/4 cup honey (or sugar substitute)
- 1 tablespoon lemon juice

Instructions:

1. Combine the mixed berries, honey, and lemon juice in a blender.
2. Blend until smooth.
3. Pour the mixture into a shallow dish and freeze for 2-3 hours.
4. Every 30 minutes, use a fork to fluff the sorbet to achieve a granita-like texture.
5. Serve the berry sorbet for a refreshing treat.

Chocolate Avocado Mousse

Ingredients:

- 2 ripe avocados
- 1/4 cup cocoa powder
- 1/4 cup honey (or sugar substitute)
- 1/2 teaspoon vanilla extract

Instructions:

1. Scoop the avocado flesh into a blender.
2. Add cocoa powder, honey, and vanilla extract.
3. Blend until the mixture is smooth and creamy.
4. Refrigerate for at least 30 minutes before serving. Garnish with berries or nuts if desired.

Rice Pudding with Raisins

Ingredients:

- 1 cup cooked white rice
- 2 cups milk (or a milk substitute)
- 1/4 cup raisins
- 1/4 teaspoon ground cinnamon
- 1/4 teaspoon vanilla extract

- 2 tablespoons sugar (or sugar substitute)

Instructions:

1. In a saucepan, combine the cooked rice and milk.

2. Add raisins, cinnamon, vanilla extract, and sugar.

3. Cook over low heat, stirring frequently, until the mixture thickens.

4. Remove from heat and let it cool. Serve chilled.

Peach and Almond Crumble

Ingredients:

- 4 cups sliced peaches (fresh or frozen)
- 1/2 cup almond meal
- 1/4 cup rolled oats
- 2 tablespoons honey (or sugar substitute)
- 1/4 teaspoon almond extract

Instructions:

1. Preheat your oven to 350°F (175°C).

2. In a baking dish, arrange the sliced peaches.

3. In a separate bowl, combine almond meal, rolled oats, honey, and almond extract.

4. Sprinkle the almond-oat mixture over the peaches.

5. Bake for 25-30 minutes until the crumble is golden brown.

6. Serve warm with a dollop of yogurt or a scoop of frozen yogurt.

Chia Seed Pudding

Ingredients:

- 1/4 cup chia seeds
- 1 cup milk (or a milk substitute)
- 1 tablespoon honey (or sugar substitute)
- 1/2 teaspoon vanilla extract
- Mixed berries for topping

Instructions:

1. In a container, mix chia seeds, milk, honey, and vanilla extract.

2. Stir well and cover. Refrigerate for at least 4 hours or overnight.

3. Before serving, top with mixed berries for added flavor and color.

Frozen Yogurt with Berries

Ingredients:

- 2 cups plain yogurt (or Greek yogurt)
- 1/4 cup honey (or sugar substitute)
- 1 cup mixed berries (strawberries, blueberries, raspberries)

Instructions:

1. In a bowl, combine yogurt and honey.
2. Freeze the mixture in an ice cream maker according to the manufacturer's instructions.
3. Serve the frozen yogurt with fresh mixed berries on top.

Watermelon and Mint Salad

Ingredients:

- 4 cups cubed watermelon
- 2 tablespoons fresh mint leaves, chopped
- 1 tablespoon lime juice

Instructions:

1. In a large bowl, combine the cubed watermelon and chopped mint leaves.
2. Drizzle with lime juice and gently toss to combine.
3. Refrigerate for a refreshing and hydrating dessert.

Banana Ice Cream

Ingredients:

*   4 ripe bananas
*   1/4 cup plain yogurt (or a yogurt substitute)
*   1 tablespoon honey (or sugar substitute)

Instructions:

1. Peel and slice the bananas.
2. Freeze the banana slices for a few hours or until firm.
3. In a blender, combine the frozen banana slices, yogurt, and honey.
4. Blend until smooth and creamy.
5. Serve immediately as a guilt-free banana ice cream.

Pistachio Biscotti

Ingredients:

- 1 cup shelled pistachios
- 1 1/2 cups all-purpose flour
- 1/2 cup sugar (or sugar substitute)
- 1/2 teaspoon baking powder
- 1/4 teaspoon salt
- 2 large eggs
- 1/2 teaspoon vanilla extract

Instructions:

1. Preheat your oven to 325°F (160°C).
2. In a bowl, combine flour, sugar, baking powder, and salt.
3. In a separate bowl, whisk together eggs and vanilla extract.
4. Add the wet ingredients to the dry ingredients and mix until you have a dough.
5. Fold in the pistachios.
6. Form the dough into two logs on a baking sheet.
7. Bake for 20-25 minutes until the logs are golden.

8. Slice into biscotti cookies and bake for an additional 10 minutes until they're crispy.

Mixed Berry Parfait

Ingredients:

- 1 cup mixed berries (strawberries, blueberries, raspberries)
- 1 cup Greek yogurt (or yogurt substitute)
- 2 tablespoons honey (or sugar substitute)

Instructions:

1. In a glass or bowl, layer Greek yogurt, mixed berries, and a drizzle of honey.
2. Repeat the layers.
3. Top with an extra sprinkle of berries and honey for a visually appealing dessert.

Oatmeal Cookies

Ingredients:

- 1 1/2 cups rolled oats
- 1/2 cup whole wheat flour

- 1/2 teaspoon baking soda

- 1/4 teaspoon salt

- 1/2 cup unsweetened applesauce

- 1/4 cup honey (or sugar substitute)

- 1/4 cup chopped dried apricots

- 1/4 cup chopped nuts (e.g., almonds or walnuts)

Instructions:

1. Preheat your oven to 350°F (175°C).
2. In a bowl, combine oats, whole wheat flour, baking soda, and salt.
3. In another bowl, mix applesauce and honey.
4. Combine the wet and dry ingredients, then add apricots and nuts.
5. Drop spoonfuls of dough onto a baking sheet.
6. Bake for 12-15 minutes until they're lightly browned.

Carrot Cake Bites

Ingredients:

- 2 cups grated carrots

- 1/2 cup chopped dates

- 1/2 cup chopped nuts (e.g., walnuts or almonds)

- 1/2 teaspoon ground cinnamon

- 1/4 teaspoon ground nutmeg

- 1/4 teaspoon vanilla extract

Instructions:

1. In a food processor, combine grated carrots, dates, nuts, cinnamon, nutmeg, and vanilla extract.

2. Process until the mixture forms a sticky dough.

3. Roll the dough into bite-sized balls.

4. Refrigerate for about 30 minutes before serving.

Pineapple Upside-Down Cake

Ingredients:

- 1 can of pineapple slices in juice (reserve the juice)

- 1/2 cup whole wheat flour

- 1/2 cup sugar (or sugar substitute)

- 1/2 teaspoon baking powder

- 1/4 teaspoon salt

- 1/4 cup unsweetened applesauce

- 1 egg

- Maraschino cherries for garnish (optional)

Instructions:

1. Preheat your oven to 350°F (175°C).
2. Arrange pineapple slices in a greased cake pan, placing a cherry in the center of each slice.
3. In a bowl, combine whole wheat flour, sugar, baking powder, and salt.
4. Mix in reserved pineapple juice, applesauce, and egg.
5. Pour the batter over the pineapple slices.
6. Bake for 30-35 minutes until a toothpick comes out clean.
7. Invert the cake onto a plate so the pineapple is on top.

Pumpkin Pie

Ingredients:

- 1 prepared graham cracker crust
- 1 cup canned pumpkin puree
- 1/2 cup milk (or a milk substitute)
- 1/4 cup sugar (or sugar substitute)
- 1/2 teaspoon ground cinnamon
- 1/4 teaspoon ground nutmeg
- 1/4 teaspoon ground ginger
- 1/4 teaspoon vanilla extract

- 2 eggs

Instructions:

1. Preheat your oven to 375°F (190°C).
2. In a bowl, combine pumpkin puree, milk, sugar, cinnamon, nutmeg, ginger, vanilla extract, and eggs.
3. Mix until smooth.
4. Pour the mixture into the graham cracker crust.
5. Bake for 40-45 minutes until set.
6. Let it cool before slicing and serving.

Angel Food Cake with Berries

Ingredients:

- 1 store-bought angel food cake
- 2 cups mixed berries (strawberries, blueberries, raspberries)
- 1/4 cup sugar (or sugar substitute)
- 1 cup whipped topping (or whipped yogurt)

Instructions:

1. Slice the angel food cake into individual servings.
2. In a bowl, mix mixed berries and sugar.

3. Top each slice of angel food cake with mixed berries
    and a dollop of whipped topping.

Caramelized Bananas

Ingredients:

- 2 ripe bananas
- 2 tablespoons brown sugar (or sugar substitute)
- 1/4 cup unsalted butter (or butter substitute)
- 1/4 cup rum (optional)
- Vanilla ice cream (or a dairy-free alternative)

Instructions:

1. In a skillet, melt the butter over medium heat.
2. Add brown sugar and stir until it caramelizes.
3. Add sliced bananas and sauté until they're tender.
4. Add rum (if using) and ignite for a flambe effect (be
    cautious).
5. Serve the caramelized bananas over a scoop of
    vanilla ice cream.

Chocolate-Dipped Strawberries

Ingredients:

- 12 fresh strawberries
- 4 ounces dark chocolate (70% cocoa or higher)

Instructions:

1. Melt the dark chocolate in a microwave-safe bowl in 20-second intervals, stirring between each, until smooth.
2. Dip each strawberry into the melted chocolate, covering it partially.
3. Place the dipped strawberries on a parchment paper-lined tray.
4. Refrigerate until the chocolate sets.

CONCLUSION

In this final chapter, we're not just saying goodbye but paving the way for your continued success. We also offer our heartfelt words of encouragement. Changing your dietary habits can be challenging, but it's worth it.

We want you to know that you're not alone in this journey. Many individuals have embarked on this path, and they've not only managed their kidney health but have also discovered a newfound appreciation for delicious, nourishing meals.

The Conclusion chapter is a reminder that, while this cookbook may be coming to an end, your renal diet journey is just beginning. Your health is an ongoing story, and the choices you make each day can contribute to a happier, healthier future.

It's a journey marked by resilience, growth, and self-care, and we applaud you for taking that first step. So, as you read the final chapter, remember that you have the tools, knowledge, and support to thrive on your renal diet path. Your story is just beginning, and we're here to cheer you on every step of the way.